Common Sense Medicine

COMMON SENSE MEDICINE:

RESTORING THE PATIENT/ PHYSICIAN RELATIONSHIP

By Jeff Danby

Alethos Press – St Paul, MN

COMMON SENSE MEDICINE:
RESTORING THE PATIENT/PHYSICIAN RELATIONSHIP
By Jeff Danby

ISBN 978-0-9849552-2-0

Copyright © 2016: Jeff Danby

All rights reserved. No reproduction in all or in part in any form is authorized without written permission. Permission is granted to quote any portion of this book with proper citation.

ALETHOS PRESS – St Paul MN

Printed in the U.S.A. by Bethany Press International
Bloomington, MN

Edited by Dave Racer, MLitt

Second Printing

TABLE OF CONTENTS

Do you care? — 1

Why doesn't medical care operate the same way as everything else in life? — 3

Why don't we have price discovery in medicine? — 8

Shouldn't we demand that the government simply fix the problem? — 12

Why can't the government simply "regulate" the current system better? — 15

How is it "harmful" for government to expand powers beyond the role of a "referee"? — 17

How and why are regulatory agencies "captured"? — 18

But isn't medical care a "basic human right"? — 21

Where is medical care a "right," and where does it become "armed robbery"? — 24

Medical care is a basic necessity of life. Shouldn't we make an exception? — 26

What if purchasing food was like purchasing medicine? — 29

Common Sense Medicine

What about catastrophic events?	35
Some people are "uninsurable" or cannot afford catastrophic health insurance!	35
Final thought: Medical care is about more than money.	36
Sacred Bonds.	39
SUMMARY	42
How to become an empowered patient and an empowered citizen.	45
GLOSSARY	50
The "Classic" Oath of Hippocrates	53
Further reading	55
About the author	56
To order more copies	57

Where is the Life we have lost in living?
Where is the wisdom we have lost in knowledge?
Where is all the knowledge we have lost in information?

~ T.S. Eliot

Common Sense Medicine

Do you care?

Let me ask you this simple question: *Are you happy with the current medical system or do you want one that is far more efficient and delivers the greatest benefits to all?*

Take a moment and ponder the question. If you don't care about problems in our medical system, then this book is not for you. Put it down and go do something else. You are irrelevant to the rest of us who demand a better way.

If you don't see any problems, then you must be living in a dream world. Perhaps you live the charmed life of a U.S. Senator or Representative, with a pool of taxpayers and a central bank paying for everything you could ever want. You do not have to worry about a person's personal costs or budgets—at least not for the time being. Life is wonderful for you, I suppose. Although the rest of us may fantasize at times about living in your shoes, we know that everybody simply cannot live at the expense of everybody else. Nothing would ever get done and all of humanity would end up either dirt poor or dead. In the end, *somebody* has to do the work. Products must be made first before they can be exchanged for other goods or services. A smiling Member of Congress or charismatic President might excite and seduce us during an election year into believing in "free lunches," Santa Claus giveaways, or redistributive "utopias," but deep down many of us realize that real life does not and cannot operate this way—at least not for the 99 percent.

If you've stuck with me this far, then we probably share similar insights on human nature and a common concern over the direction of American medical care. I am assured that you are ***not*** a U.S. Congressman. If you were, you would have tossed this essay aside by now and headed for the nearest TV camera to keep your personal gravy train a-rolling.

The good news is that we can reason our way through this medical care mess together—without the unwelcome intrusion of a blow-hard politician, condescending President, or even the United States Supreme Court. By using analogies, investigating well-known economic laws, and untangling this problem one knot at a time, we can rediscover the simple key to successful and lasting reform of American medical care. I promise the process won't take long, and the solution will not be difficult to apply. I truly believe that no matter where you fall along the political spectrum, we will both end up agreeing far more than we disagree. I believe that most of us really want the same things and should not feel frustrated, isolated, or defensive about our hopes and aspirations for society—even though certain interests vested in keeping the current unworkable system try their darndest to keep us divided and believing otherwise. Good medicine is not a left vs right, north vs south, or red vs blue issue. Good medicine is just good medicine!

Come! Join the growing chorus of medical consumers who demand the lowest medical costs along with the widest range of care choices, and we will achieve it in the end!

Why doesn't medical care operate the same way as everything else in life?

Have you ever wondered why you can almost always set up an appointment with a barber, veterinarian, or even an auto mechanic the *same day* you phone, but often must wait *weeks* to see a doctor? You should be able to see your doctor just as quickly, right? Don't you also hate that an unsympathetic insurance company or an impersonal government bureaucracy can force you to see *their* doctor when you prefer the care of another? You can choose any veterinarian, dentist, tattoo artist, or manicurist you want without some authoritarian outsider bossing you around. Why should a doctor be different? You don't have to settle for this!

Why are you also forced to complete a clipboard full of endless, confusing, and redundant paperwork before each medical visit only to suffer through months of endless, confusing, and redundant claim billings after seeing your doctor? Does your hairdresser put you through hand-cramping writing marathons like this? Does your dentist, chiropractor, yoga instructor, or gym trainer lecture you about seatbelt use, or prod you over how much alcohol or tobacco you consume, or ask you whether you own a firearm? If your massage therapist began interrogating you about your sexual history, wouldn't you bolt for the nearest exit? These non-physician "healthcare" professionals would never ask such creepy questions unless your responses were directly related to the reason for your visit.

What makes your medical doctor any different? Perhaps you simply want your M.D. to examine your wrist to see if it is broken. Why then, do you have to also endure blood pressure tests, weight checks, and lectures about colonoscopies, blood cholesterol, and smoking cessation? Why all the stupid, irrelevant questions and time-wasting measures? When you want to explain yourself to your doctor do you feel he or she is even *listening* to you? It's as if your M.D. is reading from someone else's script. Perhaps she is! Is this acceptable to you? Do you ever wonder to whom she's reporting your responses and how it might be used against you later? Do you realize that your doctor is being forced to spy on you just to be paid for treating you? Do you want to be blacklisted as "non-compliant" because you choose not to answer, or do you want your physician driven into retirement for refusing to participate in such nonsense? This is exactly what's happening across the country.

Finally, why can't you ever get a straight answer about the cost of your medical care when you call the number on the back of your insurance card? What if your credit card worked the same way the medical care system does? What if you were never sure which of your department store purchases were "covered" or "non-covered" by your bank? What if you had to "pre-authorize" all large purchases—and still weren't sure how a "deductible" would be applied? What if you had to wait for weeks and months for all those credit card charges to trickle in and ended up being threatened with 30, 60, and 90-day delinquency notices for purchases you did not make, do not recognize, or thought were "covered"? Imagine the mess—what a ridiculous way to pay for anything!

Why then do we tolerate our insane pricing system for medical care? In every other purchase you make, you always know or negotiate the price up front and shop accordingly. The process between a buyer and a seller is called ***price discovery*** and is absolutely essential for a healthy economy to function. It does not matter if a transaction is large or small—there must always be ***price discovery*** first between buyer and seller. You would never sign an agreement to buy a house without first knowing all the charges. What if you purchased a house believing the price was $100,000 and discovered later that your mortgage company charged you $500,000? I am sure you'd be hopping mad! Would you ever buy an unpriced box of nails from a hardware store on the assurance that an itemized bill would be sent later? What if you received that bill and discovered that each nail was listed at $7, the box as $25, a "stocking" fee of $15, a "check-out" fee of $12, etc.? This would be an absurdity worthier of a *Monty Python* sketch than a real life economy. Yet this is how most of our medical services are priced and we are told by straight-faced "experts" that this way "works." Perhaps this "works" for somebody, but it's not for you or your doctor. Why can't both sides simply negotiate a price *up front* like we do with everything else?

Price discovery not only eliminates confusion between a buyer and a seller, but also provides "real time" *signals* to the rest of the world of which products and services *you* prefer and how much *you* are willing to pay for them. Prices are the way consumers and suppliers *communicate* with each other. Prices are the ongoing language of an economy—just as vital as the verbal and written language we use every day to convey our wishes and desires clearly to one another. Imagine if we were not permitted to speak to each other using our own words and sentences – what terrible misunderstandings and mistakes would follow and how much poorer would society end up as a result! When we are not permitted to speak to each other with the language of *price*, terrible misunderstandings and mistakes follow and society also becomes poorer. Does this make sense to you?

Whenever you purchase something you are also "voting" for that good or service and assigning value in comparison to other available goods and services. As billions of consumer "votes" are cast daily, prices rise and fall on everything according to the sum of all those preferences. This is true "democracy" and "people power" in action! Honest consumer-driven pricing informs suppliers when to create more of one thing, less of another, or to go do something else. Prices tell Ford to make Mustangs instead of Edsels, and Apple to make iPhones instead of rotary desk phones. The processes of an economy are too fluid, unpredictable, vast, and complex for anybody to ever fully comprehend except at the most rudimentary level. This is why prices cannot be "managed" or "directed" by anybody except consumers. A famous essay called "I, Pencil" by Leonard Read cleverly illustrated that no person can ever have the full knowledge on how to build a pencil—yet pencils are ubiquitous because of this complex, "organic," and vital process we call ***natural price discovery***.

Prices are also a floating ***benchmark*** whereby suppliers must compete with *each other* for your business. Those who are able to provide more value at less cost to consumers are rewarded with more purchases. This is how Netflix came to be streamed directly into consumers' homes and Blockbuster VHS rental tapes ended up in flea market bins. This is why you have downloaded some apps onto your iPhone and not others. You choose! This phenomenon is not crazy rocket science but simply the way human beings have been successfully trading and interacting with one another for countless millennia. Everybody innately understands this. ***Price discovery*** is the essential ingredient missing in American medical care!

Why don't we have price discovery in medicine?

We don't have price discovery in medicine because the natural negotiation process between patient and doctor has been usurped slowly over time by a wide assortment of outsiders engaged in ***rent seeking***. Do not confuse ***rent seeking*** with legitimate rent collection. "Rent collection" is where an owner lends out the use of his property in exchange for money. ***Rent seeking*** is a predatory practice where an outsider siphons value out of an economic process—yet provides little or no value to the actual participants. ***Rent seekers*** are unneeded middlemen. ***Rent seeking*** almost always uses the coercive powers of government to secure guarantees for special pricing, "carve out" revenue streams, limits on competition, or even monopoly grants over some or all aspects of the process. In other words, the law is twisted to favor outsiders over consumers and suppliers. Make no mistake about it – ***rent seeking*** steals away your right to bargain with a seller and makes you a loser! Think of it as a stranger forcing his iPhone app choices on you and then overcharging you for the "service."

In medicine, these outsiders are generally ***third party vendors*** or ***agents*** who are supposed to be *serving* the needs of either the patient or the doctor. Instead, they have taken more and more *control* of decisions that rightfully belong to the only two parties that matter: the patient and doctor. These vendors and agents include insurance companies, drug companies, middlemen who process it all, and governmental regulatory agencies. Because of their ravenous and wasteful ***rent seeking*** demands, doctors have been squeezed out of attending to the needs of their patients and captured into serving these outsiders. The demands are onerous, capricious, contradictory, and demoralizing. Many doctors are quitting as a result. This causes doctor shortages and longer waits for care. Patients have been seduced and silenced into submission with false assurances that their rising medical bills will always be paid by "somebody" else, and that they are "entitled" to even more "free care." The result has been the loss of consumer control, reams of idiotic paperwork, obtrusive and irrelevant surveys, and an incomprehensible cost-shifting payment system that nobody can understand. One of the newest rages, government mandated electronic record keeping, is just a whole new layer of unnecessary ***rent seeking*** designed to impoverish the many to benefit the few.

Rent seeking may be as old as the hills but is always a counterproductive and anti-social practice. ***Rent seeking*** cripples economies because it distorts ***natural price discovery*** between the true buyer and seller. The more that honest pricing is obscured, the less suppliers are able to determine which goods and services consumers truly want and the less they can compete with each other to provide the most value at the lowest possible cost. When price distortions occur, too much of one thing is mistakenly offered and not enough of another. This is called a ***misallocation of resources*** by economists. Prices rise, shortages occur, and confusion reigns. People want less expesnive Mustangs and iPhones but are, instead, forced to settle for clunky, over-priced Edsels and "Ma Bell" landline phones—and then wait months or even years to receive them. Everyone gets mandated anchovies on their pizza whether he or she wants them or not. Everyone—other than the ***rent seeker***—ends up far poorer than he or she should be. Worse, the ***rent seekers*** use the resulting public confusion and discontent to lobby for even more government controls to "correct" the original mess that it made! This vicious cycle causes the price system to go even more haywire—leading to greater shortages, higher prices, and nastier finger-pointing over the blame. The end stage resembles rabid hyenas fighting over the remnants of a carcass. ***Rent seeking***, left unbridled, bankrupts great nations and causes entire civilizations to collapse.

Remember how we learned that prices are the vital language of an economy? Now imagine if some outsider slowly altered your verbal and written communications one word at a time so that neither you nor your associates could ever be completely sure of the other's meaning. You might still be able to get your ideas across to one another—but not without expending extra time, effort, and expense. As the outsider's interference in your communications increased, the toll on your time, effort, and expense would also rise accordingly and you would end up far less productive (and much poorer) as a result. Eventually, you would find it completely impossible to communicate at all. In the end, only the meddling outsider's words would remain—leaving you and your associates completely silenced, isolated, and suspicious of each other. This is what has happened with price communication in medicine.

The destructive effects of ***rent seeking*** are not always immediate or obvious. It can take years for price errors to build up. Sometimes an entire generation passes before anyone realizes a serious crisis is brewing. Certainly, those benefiting from price distortions will do everything they can to conceal their culpability. They play an ongoing shell game of shifting costs, shifting burdens, and shifting blame, and they will demand more outsider interference and heavier layers of control. They are, after all, gaining much from their unnecessary interference—whether that reward is a greater share of "easy" money or more draconian methods of social control. Don't be fooled. The root cause of this mess is that ***natural price discovery*** between medical buyers and sellers has been usurped by outsiders. Neither side can properly communicate with each other because of the widespread, unnecessary, and self-serving interference by outsiders. The whole reason for our "healthcare crisis" is really this simple!

Common Sense Medicine

Shouldn't we demand that the government simply fix the problem?

What do you want government to do?

If you want the government to distort *natural price discovery* even further, then you are only asking for a bigger mess. This is precisely why a "Single Payer" system can never work in the long run. Under such a scheme, government officials completely substitute *their* desires for those of both the patient and the physician. If a panel of bureaucrats was given complete control of planning everybody's meals, would you expect the country to be content with the official menu? Humans always chafe under such limits! Society would very quickly splinter apart into special interest groups and lobbies locked in bitter, never-ending battles with one another to influence what food goes on the government menu. Everybody would claw, punch and clamber over each other for the ear of some all-powerful bureaucrat. What if you hate pizza? Too bad! The pro-pizza party controls the panel. You must eat pizza on Thursday or go without food. What if you hate anchovies? Too bad! The anchovy industry has purchased more political clout then you ever can. You're taxed heavily to buy anchovies; if you don't like them you must pick them off your rationed slice! In effect, "Single Payer" forces *everybody* to become a *rent seeker* trying to curry government favors. This is precisely what makes government so dysfunctional and unpopular today. "Single Payer" would place government corruption and influence peddling on mega-steroids and be the furthest thing from *natural* pricing one could ever get!

Without *natural price discovery*, innovation also stagnates. Little incentive remains for entrepreneurs and inventors to develop new or better ways of doing anything. Nobody can even measure whether an innovation is "better" without honest pricing. Unless a government bureaucrat demands a change, nothing happens...and bureaucrats are notoriously risk-aversive, self-serving creatures. That is why bureaucrats become bureaucrats and not entrepreneurs. In fact, entrepreneurs are viewed as "enemies of the state" because their "revolutionary" ideas threaten bureaucratic authority and a stagnant social order. As entrepreneurs are silenced, the public must be forever content living in a grey world with shrinking supplies of rotary dial telephones and Blockbuster VHS rentals. As bureaucratic power increases, no one even dares to conceive of an iPhone app or a streaming Netflix.

Finally, without *natural price discovery*, the demand for medical services skyrockets. Patients and doctors can no longer *self-ration* by adjusting their expectations to natural price signals because no reliable signals exist. Nobody cares about *cost*—only about obtaining *benefits* for themselves. Putting medicine under government control will never create more medical resources. In fact, resources shrink because there is less incentive for producers to provide them. Government control does, however, simulate greater demand for those resources. To rein in demand to match an ever shrinking supply, government bureaucrats must **ration** medical resources according to their own whims. How do you convince a bureaucrat to **ration** goods and services your way? Well, how is this problem handled now? If you think well-reasoned arguments and compelling spreadsheet figures carry the day, you are dangerously naive. What happens if the bureaucrat doesn't like you personally, or finds your special interest group's petition "lacking"? Maybe you can find a way to sweeten the deal or convince some bigger bureaucrat up the chain— or perhaps not. Maybe your bureaucrat is a social engineering zealot, "social justice" disciple, or strict utilitarian, and your concerns, pitches, and bribes mean nothing to him whatsoever. Maybe he is capricious or simply crazy. Nevertheless, you had better do exactly what the medical bureaucrat tells you to do. Don't do or say anything to upset the bureaucrat!

You will not fix the delivery of medical care by eliminating buyers and sellers completely and putting a "Single Payer" in charge of everything. You will only make matters far, far worse.

Why can't the government simply "regulate" the current system better?

Government *can never know* what is better for you than you do. Everyone is a unique human being with a unique set of circumstances, desires, and needs. What works for one person might not work for another. No government official can know more about the medical arts or how to best apply this myriad of knowledge to your particular concern than your preferred doctor. If a bureaucrat knew what your doctor knows then the bureaucrat would be practicing medicine instead! Can a bureaucrat farm better than a farmer or teach better than a teacher? Can a bureaucrat build a better bridge than a structural engineer? Why would we need doctors, farmers, teachers, or engineers if bureaucrats are better at meeting our needs in those areas of expertise? The knowledge of a bureaucrat is always *less* than the consumers and producers in any economic transaction and will always be less!

The ***only*** way a government can help an economy is to remain on the periphery as an impartial referee. Any activity beyond that and government becomes a bumbling and destructive meddler. How do we know? For the simple reason that ***government is not needed for a trade to occur in the first place.*** Consumers would still seek out and pay for the advice and care of medical professionals even if there were no government. This happens all the time in places where government is weak, limited, or absent entirely. In fact, for most of American history, medicine operated exactly this way. Government is simply irrelevant to the question of whether a consumer can obtain care from a medical professional. Government is always the interloper in that relationship. When government begins dictating terms other than what the actual participants want, someone always ends up angry and frustrated. Would a baseball game be better if the umpire began changing calls to "help" one side over the other? Would you pay to see a "single player" basketball game with one referee shooting baskets for both teams while the players sat on the benches? The referee is not a player in the game, nor should the government be a "player" in medicine.

Consumers and producers "hire" government to gain some assurance that both sides can be trusted to hold up their end of the bargain. A patient wants to be assured the doctor will deliver what he promises. The doctor wants to be certain he will be paid the agreed upon fee. Both sides see the mutual benefit to having an impartial outsider referee the transaction. Neither side wants to be lied to, ripped off, or physically harmed by the other. So, for a small fee ("tax") levied on everyone, governments promise to punish anyone who lies, steals, or kills. That is all that government should do. Any actions or fees levied beyond this function and government causes more harm than good. In fact, government destroys its own credibility whenever it tries to do "too much." Government becomes the defrauder, thief or killer we all hoped to avoid in the first place. If government can't fulfill a basic "referee" function in a manner trustworthy to both sides, then the obvious question that must be asked is: *what good is government at all*?

Government must always take great care to represent the interests of *all* citizens—never favoring some citizens over others—otherwise it loses legitimacy and fails to serve as an honest broker. Do you feel that government is an honest broker now? Do you feel that government is trustworthy? Would you accept NFL officials meddling in football games the way government does in our medical lives? Of course not! For government to be useful, effective, and trustworthy in medicine, it must never behave as an agent or advocate for anybody or any favored faction. Its only concern should be the protection of all life, all property rights, and the enforcement of the justly agreed-upon contractual obligations of all participants.

How is it "harmful" for government to expand powers beyond the role of a "referee"?

Because of a phenomenon called *regulatory capture.*

Remember how a bureaucrat can never have greater expertise than a doctor, farmer, or engineer in those respective professions? The same principal applies to all other trades and industries. Bureaucrats are *always* at an information disadvantage in the fields they supposedly "regulate." Naturally, every bureaucrat wants to maintain job security, enhance prestige, and expand his agency's influence and control. If a bureaucrat simply drafted industry rules in a vacuum, he would risk ridicule and the loss of his position and reputation as an insufferable incompetent. To avoid unwelcome attention, he calls upon the ***expertise*** of industry insiders for assistance. As a result, the biggest players in any given industry end up writing and forever tweaking the very government rules that "regulate" their industry. This, in a nutshell, is why ***regulatory capture*** can never be prevented and why governments should not meddle with economies! Give up the naive notion that "good" government can ever control "bad" industries. Bureaucrats will always be outsmarted and outmaneuvered because of superior industry knowledge possessed by those they supposedly "regulate." The best way to control and weed out "bad" industries is to keep consumers and suppliers empowered with price "votes."

How and why are regulatory agencies "captured"?

Regulatory capture ***pays***. Rather than compete for customers on an open market, companies discover it is far cheaper to convince government officials to grant them exclusive favors, subsidies, or to draft regulations restricting their competition. Government is a mighty powerful ally indeed—with its army, police, courts, and prisons! A simple mathematical formula called ***return on investment*** (ROI) tells every business whether any commercial activity is worth pursuing. A company that invests a million dollars into developing a product that yields several more million dollars in profitable sales has a good ROI. You would be pleased, too, if you bought a stock for $100 and saw it double, triple or even quadruple in value a year later. But what if you could make a ***thousand times*** or even ***ten thousand times*** your investment—not by going through the trouble of developing a new product or service and competing fairly for customers, but by purchasing government power to instead capture markets and crush your competition? This is exactly what insurance companies, drug companies, and other vendors have done.

Because government officials are profoundly interested in keeping their jobs and expanding their own power and influence—they always listen to those with selfish interests. And because government officials can never understand an industry they supposedly "regulate" better than the industry players themselves, the regulations ***always*** end up being written by the biggest industry players. What is the result? Regulation grows so confusing, cumbersome, and expensive to follow, that everyone except the largest competitors are driven out of business. As competitors close up, consumer choices are severely restricted, relief in the courts is limited or barred, and people are even forced to purchase products they don't want (mandated coverages, vaccines, etc.). Concerning the practice of medicine, independent physicians are forced to either quit or join gargantuan, soul-crushing hospital groups. All of this drives up costs, lowers quality, reduces access, and actually makes the average consumer *sicker*.

You cannot stop *regulatory capture* by passing laws against it. Government officials are always risk averse and too keen on maintaining their jobs and increasing their own authority and influence. Commercial interests are always looking for the greatest *return on investment*. In the end, government and commercial special interests will work around any law to find common cause—to the detriment of the public good. The best way to prevent these forces from ever getting together is to stop believing in their false promises to begin with. Insist instead, that consumers and producers always engage in direct *natural price discovery*—without the manipulation of *rent seeking* outsiders. Insist that this condition is non-negotiable. Insist that the government remain only an impartial referee in all economic transactions.

All economic jargon aside, have you ever heard the old adage "too many cooks spoil the broth?" The medical system has far too many cooks fumbling about the kitchen with their own agendas and ruining the order that you (the patient) would like to place with your master chef (the doctor). As more and more cooks pile in to "fix" the nauseating broth

Common Sense Medicine

that's brewing, an even bigger mess results. It is time to throw all the cooks out of the kitchen until only the master chef and the customer remain!

But isn't medical care a "basic human right"?

First, we have to understand what a ***right*** is. Rights do not come from other human beings or institutions. A right is something everybody has because of being human. Every person has the right to life, property, and the freedom of movement, trade, and association. These are examples of some basic rights that are "inalienable"—in other words, they cannot be separated from you by anybody else. Rights can only be violated, never given or taken away. Murder is wrong because it violates the right to life. Theft is wrong because it violates the right of property. Making murder or theft "legal" would not "take away" rights of life and property—but would *violate* those rights. Slavery is wrong because it violates both the property rights and the freedom of one person to trade his or her own labor with another person or entity. It is also a serious rights violation to imprison a group of people because of their ethnic heritage, or prohibit a darker skinned man from marrying a lighter skinned woman. Notice how a ***right*** places no obligation on another except one of "non-interference." Your right to life, property, and freedom of trade, movement, and association demands nothing from me except that I leave you alone—and vice versa. If I am forced to do anything more

Common Sense Medicine

for you—for example, give you a back rub whenever you demand one—then my rights are violated. A right can also be defined as the boundary that exists between the equal interests of both you and me. Judge Andrew Napolitano sums up rights best by stating, "My right to extend my arm ends where your nose begins."

Notice that several of the rights listed in the previous paragraph have been systematically violated in the past by bad laws and supported by even worse Supreme Court decisions. Other rights continue to be violated today. When Dred Scott, a man simply seeking to reclaim his freedom to move, associate, and trade his own labor, was forced back onto a southern plantation in 1857, his rights were violated, even though the United States Supreme Court said at the time they were not. When agents of the United States government rounded up Japanese Americans during WWII and forced them to sell their business and most of their possessions, and then placed them in concentration camps, their rights were violated – even though the Supreme Court said at the time they were not. Because we clearly see the Court's errors in these decisions today, we tacitly admit that rights cannot be "granted" or revoked by one group of people over another. Rights are timeless. Rights are either recognized or violated—but never given or taken away.

Never confuse rights with ***privileges***! Beware of rent

seekers or power grabbers who deliberately blur the two concepts for their own gain. The key to understanding a *privilege* is that only the owner of a property can grant one. If I own a car, I can grant you the privilege to drive it and may prohibit the same to others. If I do not own the car to begin with, I cannot grant you or anybody else the privilege to drive it. Ownership must be a precondition before dispensing a privilege. A *right* is already "inalienable" ownership.

You and I have a basic right to go out and purchase coffee. Nobody can deny us this right. You do not, however, have a right to "free" coffee, or a right to force me to fetch and pay for your coffee. Your *right* to coffee ends where my *rights* to manage my own time and money begin. You may appeal to my sense of *charity* and ask me to purchase a cup of coffee for you, but the decision is mine, not yours. It is not *charity* if you persuade an armed police officer to force me to buy coffee for you or anyone else—even if you are "destitute" and coffee-deprived. This is NEVER acceptable, even if a majority vote of coffee drinkers agree and the US Supreme Court concurs. Forcing me to buy your coffee is armed robbery buried in euphemistic terminology. The awful truth is that you are attempting to take ownership of me and claim *privileges* to my time, labor, and property. This is the mindset of a slaveholder!

Common Sense Medicine

Where is medical care a "right" and where does it become "armed robbery?"

You and I have a basic right to go out and purchase medical care. Nobody can deny us this right. You do not have the right to "free" care, nor can you force others to provide it to you. The coffee analogy works in the exact same way. Your rights ***always*** end where mine begin, and vice versa—in ***all*** our interactions. Convincing a government to declare otherwise changes nothing. If a government ruled that all doctors had a right to a "free" paycheck whether they worked or not and everybody else had to cough up the cash to pay MDs or face imprisonment, you would rightfully call that "legalized armed robbery." It is no different for you to claim a "right" to "free" care from a doctor or your fellow citizens. Somebody else is being threatened and robbed to pay for it.

If Congress passed a law today prohibiting red-haired people from obtaining medical care, I'm certain you would consider that law a grave injustice. Obviously, a whole class of people is being denied the right to contract for an economic service. But the evil of the law is far more insidious and dangerous: the government is implying ***ownership*** of the skills of all doctors and the wishes of all patients and then attempting to confer ***privileges*** based upon these false claims of ownership. This key detail is missed by most people. If such a terrible law were passed, I am sure that many people would take

Common Sense Medicine

to the streets to demand the government "give back the rights" to red-haired people." Do you see the flaw in the demand? People are unwittingly agreeing to government's ownership claims! The better demand would be for the government to "stop claiming ownership over people and treating rights as privileges."

Government can never make claims of ownership on anybody whatsoever. Any such act is morally illegitimate—even if a majority of citizens approve and Supreme Court justices concur. You and I cannot claim ownership over other people in our private lives; therefore, we cannot delegate such a power to government officials either!

When a government forces you to buy health insurance you do not want (as with the "Affordable Care Act" or the Medicare Tax), they are *claiming ownership* of **you**. When a government dictates fees or forces doctors to ask questions or prescribe remedies they find objectionable, they are *claiming ownership* of the **doctor**. When a government restricts your choice of physician it is *claiming ownership* over both you and your doctor. Do you like being "owned" by the government? If you think it's absurd to suggest that a government would ever deny medical care for "red-haired people," then substitute the term "advanced elderly" instead. There have recently been quiet and persistent whispers among our academia and bureaucratic classes of euthanizing those they consider "drains" on the "global" medical budget. This is inevitable under a "Single Payer system" because of the rationing reasons we have already covered. Keep in mind that you and I will have little say over who will be defined as a "drain." Why? We were scammed into surrendering ownership of ourselves and will not be allowed to claim it back!

The public has been deliberately confused over the true meaning of rights, privileges, and charity. Not only has natural price discovery been compromised, but our language has as well. We can no longer speak to each other with honest prices or clear words because both forms of communication have been manipulated and corrupted by rent-seeking marketers and power-grabbing politicians. As a result, we feel bewildered, divided, defeated, and powerless.

The good news is that just recognizing this and refusing to play along can break the bad spell. That is what this book is all about!

Medical care is still a basic necessity of life. Shouldn't we make an exception?

It is true that medical care is more "necessary" to life then coffee, Edsels, or iPhones — certainly, people could live without these things longer than they could without medical care. Nevertheless, *medical care follows the same laws of supply and demand as everything else*. This is an inescapable truth. Modern medicine is comprised of a vast variety of goods and services that must still be produced with incurred costs. The wide variety of medical services available to us requires physicians to practice highly technical skills that take many years to acquire. Government cannot command medical care into existence any more than it can declare everyone instantly cured of all illnesses and be given life expectancies of 125 years. If government could command such things into existence, I would be the first to demand that I be given a free starship *Enterprise* complete with crew! To prove I am unselfish, I would demand the government provide free warp-drive starships and crews to *everybody*!

All that government can ever hope to do is redistribute goods and services that already exist—and must make continual threats of fines, imprisonment, and violence in order to do so. Not only are these evil and barbarous acts based upon immoral claims of ownership over people, labor and property, but the entire exercise is completely counterproductive. Forced redistribution always *destroys* value because the incentive to create future value is ruined. Why produce something useful if it's only going to be taken away from you? In fact, you're a fool to create anything at all. You're better off just sitting back, taking it easy, and waiting for government to grant you "your" share of the spoils. Fostering a perverse economic incentive like this does nothing to help the poor. Instead, forced redistribution causes the vast majority to become far *poorer*. Of course, the bureaucrats wielding the power to redistribute never suffer. As the economic pie shrinks and living standards plummet for everybody else, government re-distributers always find ways to pay themselves and their closest cronies handsomely and to blame scapegoats for the damage. Who can stop them? They control the army, the police, the courts, the prisons, the media, and now "own" you and anything you create!

Even after all this evidence, if you still believe that government must be more than a "referee" because medicine is a "basic necessity," let's try one more little thought exercise. Let's imagine how another "basic necessity" might be ruined if it was meddled with and abused as poorly as medicine is today.

Let's look at ***food***.

Food is even more essential to human life than medical care. Without medical care, many people can still live a long life lasting for several decades or more. Without food, *everybody* dies in only a matter of weeks. Yet, most of us have no trouble obtaining food when we want or need it. This is because **natural price discovery** between buyer and seller has not been destroyed in regards to food. As a result, in the United States, food is plentiful and relatively inexpensive. It can be found virtually everywhere: grocery stores, restaurants, and even gas stations. You are free to choose where you purchase your food. If you do not like the price or quality offered in one place, you can go down the street and purchase it somewhere else. If you do not want to wait for a table at one restaurant, you may find another where you will be immediately seated. You vote with your feet and with your money about where you will purchase food and how much you are willing to pay. The choice is purely yours. No force is involved. This is true "people power" and "democracy." This is peace and civilization. This way works. This way is *better*.

What if purchasing food was like purchasing medicine?

What if you had no idea how much your food cost, and the grocer or restaurant menu could not tell you at the time of service? What if you had to submit claims every single time you made a food purchase and then wait weeks to find out what was covered or not covered?

What if government forced you to buy expensive "food insurance" or enroll in "Bronze," "Silver," or "Gold" "food exchange" programs? What if you risked IRS penalties for failing to do so? What if, upon turning 65-years old, you were forced to join "Meal-icare" and not allowed to buy food, and your "Meal-icare Provider" was not allowed to sell you food outside the program? What if many food providers stopped taking "Meal-icare" out of frustration over unreliable reimbursements and because of layer upon layer of contradictory bureaucratic demands?

What if your "food policy" included expensive mandated coverage for foods that you will never eat but are still forced to buy because the government determined they were "good for you?" What if you were a conscientious vegetarian or lactose intolerant but were still forced to subsidize "free" meat and dairy products for everybody else? What if your children were made to ingest questionable "vitamins" pushed by powerful pharmaceutical companies or face expulsion from school?

What if more exotic or expensive food purchases had to be "pre-authorized" and your requests were often denied as "unnecessary," "experimental," or an "over-utilization"? What if the FDA ruled organic foods were "quackery" and your policy only paid for the overpriced, bland, processed fare churned out by gargantuan agri-businesses in bed with government regulatory agencies? What if farmers' markets were forced out of business and gobbled up by those same enormous agri-businesses as the result of prohibitive compliance costs. What if the complaints of small farmers fell on deaf ears? What if every food supplier was forced to maintain expensive "electronic records" to report on all their customers' purchases, and had to pay for "food malpractice" policies costing tens of thousands of dollars, and had to employ staffs of full-time "food coding" specialists to file claims for reimbursements? What if only the few "Big Farma" firms that wrote the rules could afford to follow them—but whenever they broke a rule themselves, were only given a "slap on the wrist." What if you could sue a small farmer out of business, but damages were "capped" or lawsuits were too expensive to adjudicate if you tried to sue "Big Farma"? What if you were not allowed not sue "Meal-icare" at all?

What if you had to make a grocery store appointment for bread weeks ahead of time and then book a new appointment for milk weeks later because your "food provider" was not allowed to "bundle" sales in one visit? What if, during each visit, your grocer was required to record your weight, social security number, and question you about your salt, sugar and alcohol use, document the number of kitchen knives you own, and report all this to government bureaucrats?

What if you had to obtain a "prescription" for meat and then visit a separate butcher across town to have the order filled? What if your "protein prescriptions" were denied beyond an "allowable" 30-day supply?

What if large employers were forced to provide "food insurance" for all their full-time employees and given tax breaks that were not extended to you? What if you were afraid to find another job or travel overseas for fear that your "food coverage" would not follow you? What if your company downgraded your job from full time to part time to escape skyrocketing "food insurance" costs? What if you then lost your job to a robot because robots don't require expensive government-mandated "food insurance" at all?

I think you get the picture.

This government-mandated and controlled food "system" would be an absolute nightmare, wouldn't it? There would be no end to waste, fraud, and abuse. Imagine how expensive food would become, how much worse the quality would be, and how difficult it would be to obtain. Imagine how much *worse* the poor would suffer. This is certainly *not* an efficient way to deliver a "basic necessity" in life. Yet this is *exactly* how the horror show of our current medical system works. The only thing more absurd than this "system" is the fact we actually put up with it!

There is an easier way. It works with food. It works with everything else.

It is **cash**.

Cash restores **natural price discovery**. Cash makes your personal wishes known and forces your doctor to serve *only* you. Cash is king. Cash restores "people power." Cash restores sanity.

Cash works NOW in medical services that are offered outside our insane system. Wherever these services are subjected to open and competitive pricing, prices come down dramatically. Lasik eye surgery and cosmetic procedures are prime examples. "Cash pay" medical clinics and surgery centers are beginning to pop up all across the United States because patients and doctors alike are sick of all the hassles and high prices inherent to the government-designed and mandated medical care system. These cash businesses are able to offer medical services, procedures, and surgeries at a *fraction* of current costs simply by cutting out all the ***rent-seeking*** middlemen.

"Cash pay" centers are also flourishing outside the control of US and other nations that have "socialized medicine" for similar reasons. Belize, India, Singapore, and Thailand all have a thriving "***medical tourist***" industry catering to foreigners who do not want to suffer or die while waiting in line for government rationed care. If there is a powerful argument against "Single Payer," this is it! As with the restaurant that gives rotten service, these medical tourists are voting with their feet!

People need ***cash*** in order to escape our rotten medical system. That cash could be freed up by allowing everyone to simply "opt out" of all government mandates, and to extend the same tax advantages to ***everybody*** that employers now receive when they purchase health insurance for their employees. Instead of those tens of billions dollars flowing into the pockets of powerful rent-seeking interests and various government busybodies, power would return to the pockets of "the people" so that every person could "vote" directly on where his or her medical dollar was to go. The power of *natural price discovery* would be unleashed, prices would drop, quality would rise and the consumer would, once again, be "king"—just like we already are when we purchase food, housing, entertainment, transportation, cell-phone service, LCD TVs, haircuts, veterinarian services and every other product and service in life.

Centrally controlled "top down" medicine does not work. Let's go in the opposite direction. Make American medical care a "320 million payer" system. Stop believing the lies pushed by rent seekers and power grabbers who tell you that medical care does not require natural price discovery, does not follow the same economic laws of supply and demand as everything else, and that you are always "entitled" to someone else's paycheck. Stop believing that bureaucrats, crony capitalists or socialist authoritarians know what's best for you or have your best interests at heart. Stop believing that "healthcare" is somehow "different."

Demand that your cash be returned as *your cash* so you and *you alone* may "vote" on where you want to spend it.

What about catastrophic events? People don't have expensive catastrophic "food" events like they do with medical care.

Catastrophic health insurance is the answer then. You do not purchase fire insurance for your house to pay for new wall paint, updated kitchens, carpet cleaning, or to replace broken light bulbs. If you did, "catastrophic" fire insurance would quickly become unaffordable. For the same reason, people do not purchase auto insurance to pay for gasoline, oil changes, or tire rotations.

If people truly fear that a catastrophic medical event might wipe them out financially, let them purchase insurance that *only covers that possibility*—the same way fire, accident or life insurance currently covers homes and autos, and financially protects families from unexpected death. If government wants to help, allow ***everyone*** to fully deduct those insurance premiums—not just employers and labor unions.

Some people are "uninsurable" or cannot afford catastrophic "health insurance"!

Some people cannot afford food, homes, autos, or other basic necessities in life *either*. This is where ***charity*** comes in. We do not toss out ***natural price discovery*** for the entire country just because some of us are hungry, homeless, or down on our luck. We provide *charity* to those less fortunate. Even government assistance programs such as "Food Stamps" or "Social Security" do not attempt to usurp natural price discovery or dictate supply and demand. Social Security checks, EBT cards, and rent assistance are distributed in the form of *cash* so that recipients still make their *own* decisions on how best to spend the money. If you strongly believe that government must provide a "safety net" for medical care, why don't you allow people shop around for catastrophic insurance or medicine the way they already do with any other product or service? Why do you support ugly paternalism when it comes to the practice of medicine? Isn't it better and far more humane to give the truly needy some monetary assistance and allow them to make their own financial decisions? If government wants to help, then government should allow everyone to fully deduct all charitable giving from their income taxes.

A final thought: Medical care is about much more than money.

Each of us is born into this world with a finite amount of time. We spend that time interacting with countless others in mutually beneficial ways. Some relationships are strictly economic ones: a good or service is exchanged without any emotional connections whatsoever. You might purchase a newspaper from a street vendor whom you never see again, or you may hire a tow truck driver to fix a flat tire and then send you on your way. However, many other "economic" interactions are far more complex and multifaceted. Although they still involve exchanges of goods, labor or information, they are not strictly "economic" relationships.

Perhaps the same barber has cut your hair for 20 years. Why? Can't you cut your own hair and save time and money? Won't any barber do? Do your haircuts involve something *more* than the mere exchange of money for labor? We all have a favorite teacher from our childhood. What made that teacher so great to you? I'm willing to bet it wasn't because he or she read dull information to you from a required text book. A popular 1980s TV comedy called *Cheers* centered on the same group of patrons meeting every evening in a Boston bar. Were these characters drawn to the beer or something more? If *Cheers* was only about the beer, each customer would have bought a six-pack for much less at a convenience store and gone home to drink alone. Why would anyone watch a show about barflies sitting around and drinking beer anyway? It's because *Cheers* was about the complex and comical human relationships that arise *while* purchasing beer. That's what drew the characters back to the bar and viewers to their televisions. The drinkers exchanged "value" that could not be quantified by money.

Interactions that you don't even consider as "economic" still involve the exchange of goods, services, and time.

Think of your daily interactions with family and friends. These involve countless "economic" transfers—although you don't think of them as such. How will you "spend" time today with your children or your spouse? Although you might think of family time as "priceless," aren't your interactions ones of "mutual benefit" where something of "value" is being exchanged? How do you "spend" time with friends? Have you ever given an afternoon of physical labor helping a buddy move into a new apartment? Were you "repaid" with free refreshments and pizza? Did you share countless jokes and laughs? Did you exchange ideas, hopes and aspirations? Do you continue to learn from each other? Does your friend give you great advice on your interpersonal relationships? Do you comfort each other when your favorite sports team blows yet another season? I'm sure you both "value" your friendship beyond anything that money can buy. There is "value" there nonetheless.

If my use of economic terms to describe your family and friendships makes you uncomfortable, then I'm pleased. That's my point! "Value" cannot be reduced down to mere money, products and services. Even interactions that we think of as primarily "economic" still include unmeasurable layers of personal, emotional, and spiritual "value" that cannot be dismissed or ignored. Human beings are extremely complex creatures with deep-seeded drives for family, camaraderie, and community. Each one of us has our own subjective value scale of what is important to us. We all seek meaning and *value* in our lives in ways that are often mysterious—even to ourselves. No people's decisions on how they spend their own time or money or with whom they wish to associate should *ever* be usurped by outsiders with ulterior motives—even when it's supposedly "for your own good" or "the good of society." You are not helping the man who enjoys idle chit-chat with his barber by jamming a set of government-issued shears into his hands and telling him to go cut his own hair. You are not helping the characters on *Cheers* by sending them home with free beer. You cannot redistribute spouses, children, or friends to help those who are lonely or are childless. ***No interpersonal relationship can ever be reduced to strict economic mathematics by outsiders!*** Such crude and ignorant intrusions into peoples' lives are self-defeating and extremely destructive of individuals and society — it is anti-human behavior!

Sacred Bonds

Societies have *always* recognized that certain human relationships *must always* be left alone—otherwise civilization itself is placed in jeopardy. For millennia, the term *sacred bond* has described the special ties between a husband and wife, parent and child, priest and confessor, attorney and client, and the ***patient and doctor***. Each of these relationships involves deep and delicate bonds of trust with immeasurable *value.* They cannot be reduced to mere economic arrangements. Thus, the *value* shared in these relationships cannot be quantified, subjugated, and "redistributed." The arrogant outsider, who dares to undermine this trust and destroy this value, shatters the most basic bonds holding civilization together.

Ask your physician why he or she chose a career in medicine. Most physicians will tell you that they enjoy helping the sick get well again. Some see their work as a deep spiritual calling. To gain some insight into this mystery, read the ancient Oath of Hippocrates at the end of this booklet. Doctors began using this oath in Greece at least 2,500 years ago, and it has been solemnly recited by generations of physicians ever since. You see, doctors gain immeasurable "value" interacting with their patients, too! On average, each doctor has gone through (at minimum) *12* grueling years of college, medical school and a residency to earn the right to help you. They are not simply dispensing "healthcare" the way some street vendor might sell you newspapers. They do not enjoy being forced into serving meddling insurance companies or government bureaucrats — they *hate* them just as much as you do. They want to serve *you*. If you find a doctor who prefers serving an agenda other than yours, my advice is to immediately seek another doctor.

Patients don't want "pill dispensers," robots, or government spies for physicians. They want real "one on one" human interaction with medical experts who are dedicated to serving ***their*** needs above any others. This is why all third-party payers and bureaucrats must be driven completely out of the exam room. They are bad "bulls in a china shop" and no help at all. Remember, too, that a physician deserves an honest wage for honest work. Honest wages can only be determined through ***natural price discovery***. Honest wages cannot be paid by using dishonest methods. Stop expecting "someone else" to pick up your tab.

The patient/physician relationship has suffered terribly from the unrelenting meddling of outsiders these past 40 years. As a result, many physicians and patients have simply given up on even trying to figure out what has gone wrong. Nevertheless, we all sense we are losing something very sacred and special. Take heart! All is not lost! Whenever anything in life becomes too complicated, a great general rule of thumb is to strip that problem down to the bare essentials. Apply the KISS rule ("Keep It Simple, Stupid"). When we do this, we can plainly see medicine is about the patient and physician relationship first and foremost. Any "help" beyond that relationship is "non-essential."

It is time to toss all imposter chefs out of the kitchen. It is not too late to save medicine!

Common Sense Medicine

SUMMARY:

America's medical care is a complete mess because ***natural price discovery*** between patient and doctor has been severely undermined over time. Third parties, vendors including insurance companies, drug companies, and other ***rent-seeking*** interests have usurped the normal language of ***price*** between buyer and seller for their own gain. Government has abandoned its proper role as an honest referee for ***all residents*** to become a player in league with ***rent-seekers.*** This has allowed ***regulatory capture***, where the rules are written to favor the ***rent seekers*** and their government allies to the detriment of everyone else.

Natural price signals are necessary to coordinate supply and demand to flow in the most efficient ways possible. Prices represent true "democracy" and "people power." They are the language each of us uses to "vote" for the products and services we want. When these signals are hijacked by outside interests, the economy falters and eventually fails. Then, human misery reigns.

Centrally planned economies never work. They *always* deliver far less than what we would have had otherwise. They *always* enrich the few at the expense of the many. The United States' medical care economy is much larger than the economies of most other countries. Economies are extremely complex, organic systems—delicate latticework with countless layers balanced and rebalanced by the decisions of hundreds of millions of consumers each day. An economy behaves more like a beautiful coral reef teeming with rich, vibrant complexity than some stark grey factory churning out a basic product like pig iron. Neither a complex coral reef nor a complex human economy can be centrally planned or commanded by a panel of meddling overseers using megaphones, guns, and paddy-wagons. This is an experiment that has been tried often and utterly fails every single time.

The lives, property and decisions of consumers and producers cannot be "owned" by anybody but the consumers and producers themselves. Those who attempt to usurp this natural ownership violate the inalienable rights we each have to run our own lives, trade our own property and time, and associate with those whom we choose. These rights are not "privileges" to be given or taken away by others. Rights are ***inseparable*** from us as human beings. Not even "majority rule" can separate rights from others. My "rights" end where your rights begin.

We live in a modern society struggling to become freer in fits and starts. We are not serfs or slaves. Thanks to the Gutenberg Press of old and the Internet of new, we have unprecedented access to all the information we need to make our own informed decisions. We do not need kings, overlords, bureaucrats, czars, or masters limiting our access to information or goods and services and running our lives for us—although they keep screaming at us that we do. We now trade in a world of EBay, Uber, and Amazon. The world is undergoing a massive decentralization tsunami that is greatly empowering individual consumers, cutting out middlemen, and reducing the need for bureaucracies and governments. You can Skype or share files instantly with anyone around the world. With a keystroke click you can order anything from anywhere in the world and have it delivered to your doorstep in a matter of days. We have apps on our cellphones that provide instant information on the things that interest us. We no longer need 19th Century style government postal service monopolies to deliver information to us in the form of metered mail. It is just as archaic and stupid to believe that medical care must be delivered in a "top down" fashion. Quite frankly, this is a 1930s approach to economic problem-solving that didn't even work in the 1930s.

Medicine is no different from any other good or service. It must follow the same laws of supply and demand. Whenever we make a purchase, we "vote" with our cash. When we fear that an unforeseen event might cause catastrophic economic loss, we purchase insurance to gain peace of mind. When we are down on our luck we ask others for charity. And when we are blessed with extra money to give, we freely give aid to those in need. We can only be **charitable** when we give our *own* money to an orphanage. We become *uncharitable thieves* when we commission Al Capone to steal from others to give to the same orphanage. Know and practice the difference!

The entire root error in the United States medical care mess can be summed up in only four words:

"No natural price discovery."

But the mess can also be fixed in just four words:

"Cash, Catastrophic Insurance, Charity."

How to Become an Empowered Patient and an Empowered Citizen:

Take ownership of yourself and your own health. Do not push responsibility for yourself onto others. You own yourself and your problems. Take advantage of all the free information around you to better yourself. Become "self-educated." If you refuse to take ownership of yourself, others will take advantage of you.

Demand to know the price of everything you purchase! Ask each of your doctors to give you a list of prices whenever you visit. Fast food joints list their prices. Grocery stores mark their products with prices. Doctors and hospitals should publish all their prices as well. If you paid with cash, you can be assured those prices would be advertised. When you pay with cash, you are also empowered to shop around for the best deal.

Demand that you may see any doctor, or use any hospital or health professional that you wish. Nobody has the right to tell you with whom you may or may not associate. No government or insurance company can take this right away from you. Your freedoms of association and trade are violated because you allow others to do so.

Demand that all insurance companies, drug companies, and government agencies butt out of the patient/physician relationship. We would not stand for government meddling in the bedroom, the law office, or the church confessional the way it currently does with medicine. Government has no role in the exam room, other than to make sure no fraud or physical abuse is taking place by either party. A patient's relationship with a health insurance company or government relief program must never ensnare the doctor. Cash is cash. Whatever arrangements the patient has made with an outsider willing to cover all or part of the patient's bill is not the doctor's concern—nor should the responsibility be shoved onto the doctor to collect fees from that outsider.

Demand the freedom for anyone to "opt out" of Medicare or the Affordable Care Act at any time. FORCED participation is not only un-American, but is immoral and evil. If people prefer government-run insurance, then they should sign up and pay for it. Nobody should *ever* be forced to buy any product or service under threats of violence, property confiscation, or imprisonment – this is called "barbarism."

Demand that government allow you to exempt ALL of your medical costs from taxation. Government plays favorites by giving employers, unions, and special interests tax breaks on medical insurance that they refuse to extend to you. Government allows some people to deduct medical costs, but not others. Is this fair? This is not being an honest broker or an impartial referee for ALL citizens.

Demand that government be an honest broker for ALL citizens, not just in regards to medical care but in ALL matters.

Demand that governments and central banks stop devaluing our money by "counterfeiting" more into existence. Counterfeiting money is theft even when declared "legal" by a government to do so. Central banking monopolies are the ultimate form of rent seeking. When one group of people is given the sole power to conjure fiat money into existence with just a keystroke, then all that is needed is enough time and those people will end up owning and controlling everything. Central banking has devastated the middle class in the United States. A dollar today is worth only a tiny fraction of what it was worth 100 years ago. This has been a 97 percent tax on *all of us*. We cannot conduct business efficiently (such as purchasing medical care) when value is systematically stolen from our money. We also cannot save and pass accumulated wealth down to our children for a "better life." The "American Dream" is dying because our money is continually corrupted and debased.

Demand an end to legal tender laws. Allow all types of money to "compete." Buyers and sellers should use whatever they wish to settle a transaction—whether this is fiat dollars, bitcoin, gold backed currency, Swiss francs, beads, or pretty seashells. It is no one else's concern what others agree to use as mediums of exchange in their trades. Societies historically settle upon "the most marketable commodity" as money. Allowing this discovery process yields honest money that is "organic" and stable and cannot be monopolized by anybody.

Do not take "no" for an answer. Don't be a jerk with your demands. Simply speak truth to power. Never resort to lies or idle threats. Never damage property or resort to violence. You will often have to retreat for tactical reasons or to maintain peace, but always return making the same clear, reasonable demands.

Communicate these ideas to others. Pass this booklet around to others. Better yet, share the *ideas* you have learned from it in your own words. Real change must always come from the "bottom up."

Never be intimidated. Whenever you root out interests that are entrenched and backed by government power, you will be treated like an "enemy." You will be called every name in the book. Rent-seekers will try to intimidate you into silence. Again, simply speak truth to power. Force has limits, but the words of truth endure forever.

Common Sense Medicine

GLOSSARY:

(Impress a friend and confound a politician! These are fancy terms for things we covered and innately understand, but did not know there were words for them.)

Price discovery - The process by which buyers and sellers of a given product or service agree to make an exchange that is expressed as monetary value. The process must be ***natural*** and unhindered from outside agendas in order to work efficiently.

Rent Seeking - The impulse to increase one's own wealth without producing additional value. The easiest way to accomplish this is by using the coercive powers of government.

Monopoly – The exclusive control of a product or service through force that allows for price manipulation.

Agent - One who is authorized to act on another's behalf, but *serves* and never acts as a superior to that person.

Third party vendor- An entity that supplies goods or services to aid in a transaction between buyer and seller but is not essential to or a direct party to that transaction.

A **Right** - Inalienable qualities that each of us share equally as human beings. Rights are inseparable. Rights can neither be given nor taken away by others. Rights can only be recognized or violated. Rights can never place an obligation on another except one of "non-interference.

A **Privilege** - A privilege is not the same thing as a right. A privilege can only be conferred by the owner of a property.

Single Payer - A system whereby the government assumes complete control of the "demand" side of an economic process. This completely destroys natural price discovery, ruins economies, and ultimately impoverishes the masses.

Regulatory capture - The inevitable process where government agencies always become controlled by the very industries they were first charged with regulating. As a result, the public interest is subverted to favor the interests of the dominant players in that industry.

Return on Investment (ROI) - A percentage of profit garnered after tax, depreciation, and original investment cost is deducted. In essence, ROI is "profit" and the "profit" of a typical successful business averages somewhere in the neighborhood of 7 percent. When a business, union, or special interest purchases government powers to gain unfair advantages over competitors or to "capture" consumers, then the ROI is often *thousands of times* higher than 7 percent.

Misallocation of Resources - The inevitable results of destroying *natural price discovery* is a "mal-investment" in products or services that really are not valued by consumers. A recent example was the "housing boom" (and a necessary subsequent "bust") where more homes were built than actually needed by consumers because of *unnatural* enticements pushed by government subsidies, artificially low interest rates, and because bad risks were buried, mixed, and bundled along with good risks into unsustainable financial derivatives.

THE "CLASSIC" OATH OF HIPPOCRATES:

(5th to 4th Century B.C.)

I swear by Apollo Physician, by Asclepius, by Health, by Heal-all, and by the gods and goddesses, making them witnesses, that I will carry out, according to my ability and judgment, this oath and this indenture: To regard my teacher in this art as equal to my parents; to make him partner in my livelihood, and when he is in need of money to share mine with him; to consider his offspring equal to my brothers; to teach him this art, if they require to learn it, without fee or indenture; and to impart precept, oral instruction, and all other learning, to my sons, to the sons of my teacher, and to the pupils who have signed the indenture and sworn obedience to the physicians Law, but to none other.

I will use treatment to help the sick according to my ability and judgment, but I will never use it to injure or wrong them. I will not give poison to anyone through asked to do so, nor will I suggest such a plan. Similarly, I will not give a pessary to a woman to cause abortion. But in purity and in holiness I will guard my life and my art.

I will not use the knife on sufferers from stone, but will give place to such as are craftsmen therein. Into whatsoever houses I enter, I will do so to help the sick, keeping myself free from all intentional wrong-doing and harm, especially

Common Sense Medicine

from fornication with woman or man, bond or free. Whatsoever in the course of practice I see or hear (or even outside my practice in social intercourse) that ought never be published abroad, I will not divulge, but consider such things to be holy secrets.

Now if I keep this oath and break it not, I may enjoy honor, in my life and art, among all men for all time; but if I transgress and forswear myself, may the opposite befall me.

(Source: http://www1.umn.edu/phrm/oaaaths/oath1.html)

Further Reading:

(If you are so inclined: Each of these works is relatively short and easy to understand. All are readily found on the Internet. Some are available as free downloads.)

Economics in One Lesson, by Henry Hazlitt (approx. 200 pages)

The Law, by Frederic Bastiat (approx. 75 pages)

Anatomy of the State, by Murray N. Rothbard (approx. 50 pages)

I, Pencil, by Leonard Read, (short essay)

Common Sense Medicine

Meet the Author: Jeff Danby

Jeff received a Bachelor of Arts in History with Honors from DePaul University in 1985, and worked as a health and life underwriter for a number of years. He is married to Melinda Woofter, MD, and the two have three children.

Jeff wrote, researched, and wrote a World War II history book on a small unit action in Southern France called *The Day of the Panzer*. This work was honored as a History Book Club and Military Book Club featured selection during the summer of 2008. Jeff is currently writing another World War II work: an exhaustive two-volume history of B Company of the 756th Tank Battalion called *Men of Armor*.

Jeff maintains a website dedicated to the memory of the 756th Tank Battalion and is an expert on that unit's history. He has helped countless family members, fellow military researchers, and other contacts from around the world with their inquiries on this unit.

He has also helped several veterans secure the documentary proof they needed to receive medals they earned but were never awarded.

Jeff is a Level 4 USA Hockey coach and is deeply involved in local hockey for both youth and adult players.

Common Sense Medicine

TO ORDER COPIES OF *COMMON SENSE MEDICINE*

To order by check, make your check payable to the Association of American Physicians and Surgeons, or simply to AAPS. **Mail your check with a photocopy of this page to**:

AAPS
1601 N Tucson Blvd - Suite 9
Tucson, AZ 85716

To use a credit or debit card, call AAPS at (800) 635-1196 to place your order. The price is $3.00 each for single copies. For orders of 25 or more copies, remit $1.00 per copy.

Please send me _____ copy(ies) of *Common Sense Medicine.* I've enclosed $_____ with this order. **Please print clearly.**

NAME: _____

STREET: _____

_____

CITY _____ **ST** _____ **ZIP** _____

DAYTIME PHONE: _____

Questions? Call (800) 635-1196 or email to aaps@aapsonline.org